Lesson In Lyme

A multi-therapeutic approach to healing
chronic infections

D1636673

Ashley Boss RN, ND

Lesson In Lyme
A multi-therapeutic approach to healing
chronic infections

Published by Ashley Boss RN, ND

Cover Designed by Stephanie Meeusen

ISBN: 1987414802

Contents

Disclaimer: Ashley is not a licensed medical doctor. Any information contained in this book is not a substitute for or should be construed as medical advice. Always consult your healthcare provider before beginning any new health care regimen and do not delay necessary medical treatment due to something you have read in this book.

Preface

As I write this book, I reflect back on the last number of years. A difficult journey, striving to find solutions to my symptoms and my husband's many symptoms and health problems. I determined, after doing thousands of hours of research and studies, to pursue a degree in Doctor of Traditional Naturopathy. To follow my dreams and passions to help others with similar challenges find these answers as well. I needed a place, this book, to share the information that I have learned about Lyme disease and the many co-infections that frequently accompany it. I have a very strong desire to assist others who are struggling to find answers as the diagnosis and/or symptoms of Lyme disease can seem hopeless. I have been a Registered Nurse for the past 11 years and have worked in the medical field for the past 15 years. This training gives me a unique perspective from both conventional and natural medicine.

There have been many peaks and valleys in the last number of years, but through this all, God has been my strength and my hope. In the valleys I have grown mentally, emotionally, and spiritually. I believe things are allowed to happen in our lives for a reason, and I have turned my pain into my purpose. This has been my motto for the last few years. At times I would cry out to God and plead with Him to heal me and my husband. After an excellent sermon about God not owing us anything, including an easy life, I started to accept that being miraculously healed was not His will at that time. That's when I started to heal emotionally, prior to that I was a mess. I had to start accepting where I was at that time, and embrace it. I needed to "slow down" in life and was forced to do so because of my health. I started to find beauty in the little things. Joy in the midst of suffering and pain, finding little things to be thankful for. Praising God for His mercy in bringing me through each day. Finding hope in Christ that this world is not my home, Heaven is my forever home, and that in Heaven there will be no more pain, no more suffering, I will have a glorified body there! God uses brokenness to bring glory to His name. In the midst of this brokenness, was also the time where my faith has grown the most.

My journey started many years ago, even as a child I struggled with health challenges. These challenges continued in high school and beyond, with vaccines worsening them and culminating with Lyme and chronic infections.

I have spent many days, months and years searching for answers on what happened. At first, all I could think, was if I could do it all over again, go back to where it all went wrong (as in not get vaccinated), how different things might be. But then, I most likely wouldn't be where I am currently, I would not have completed the research I have done because of all of these challenges. I have a different mindset now than

I had even a couple of years ago. Sometimes, I find myself wishing for our old life back. In ways it would be wonderful, but I wouldn't fit into that life now. I've changed in many ways. Trials mature you, change your priorities, and open up new opportunities and thought patterns. Changes that would not have happened without the chronic infections and health challenges that we have walked through.

I cling to the fact that God has a plan, I can have all the dreams and plans that I want, but God's plan is so much better than my plans. I need to submit completely to His timing and His will, and He provides the peace that surpasses all understanding!

Acknowledgement

I would not be where I am today with my own health, philosophy, and practice without the amazing practitioners I've had the privilege of meeting.

I would especially like to thank Dr. Irestone for his guidance in our own health challenges and for being the one to put the pieces of the puzzle together. His work, his knowledge, and all he has shared with me is priceless. There have been a few notable people in my life that have had a way of challenging me, and Dr. Irestone is one of them. Asking the right questions or giving me bits and pieces of information that fill in the gaps. His experience has brought me to where I am today.

I also am thankful to have met Dr. Newburn at a training seminar and have learned so much from him as well. It was an answer to prayer to have a practitioner with a similar philosophy to stay in contact with and bounce questions off of!

I am thankful to Mary Huenink for her friendship. God has provided me with a dear friend that could understand the challenges that we have gone through. An encouragement through the shared grief and tears, but also the hope and joy of seeing God provide answers to our many needs.

I am thankful to Stephanie Meeusen for designing the cover of this book, designing my business logos, and always being ready and willing to work on my projects. Her creativity always amazes me! So thankful for her and her husband and their friendship.

I would especially like to thank my husband for supporting my return to school for my ND, being my "test subject", and being the business side of Alternative Approach Wellness Center. For being the editor of this book and all of my other written things and making sure I write in a way others can understand!

Thank you to all the other family and friends not mentioned by name. Thank you for your support in many different ways and your prayers on our behalf.

Ultimately, I thank God for leading us and opening doors in ways only He could. I am thankful He allowed Lyme to happen in my life. It has changed me in ways I cannot fully explain. So many times when things seemed humanly impossible, God made it possible and doors swung wide open!

My Story

I was diagnosed with asthma at 8 years old. The severity of this condition fluctuated over the years. Some years, there were no symptoms, other years there were symptoms just about every day. One summer, when I was around 10 years old, I remember being confined to a lawn chair for many days watching my brother and sister play outside. I wasn't able to play with them because my asthma attacks were so severe. Walking 30 feet would make me so short of breath, it would take me 10-15 minutes to recover.

I look back at other symptoms I had during high school and college years. Symptoms like bloating and abdominal pain, things I now recognize as probable GI issues or leaky gut. At the time, I didn't know these things shouldn't be "normal".

At 20 years old I received many vaccines prior to a medical mission trip to Nigeria. About a month after returning home from Africa, I developed significant nausea which lasted a few months. I lost 20 pounds in less than a month and weighed under 95 pounds for over a year. I'm 5'7", have always had fine bone structure and been thin, but this was not normal! My family doctor didn't know what was wrong with me. He basically told me I was fine and to go on and live my life. 11 years after the fact, we discovered that I have had a chronic Hepatitis A infection. This is most likely from the Hepatitis A vaccine that I received prior to the trip to Nigeria.

The following year, I would get sick with viruses, colds, flus about once every month. I found this all very strange as I had been fairly healthy overall and would usually only get sick with a minor cold once or twice a year. I had large, painful canker sores in my mouth that would come and go month after month. I now realize these were symptoms of being poisoned. Poisoned by the toxins in the vaccines, and my body was attempting to rid itself of these toxins! The asthma that was fairly stable before became much more frequent. Seasonal allergies became so severe that at times during late summer and fall I would take multiple antihistamines to get through a day without sneezing constantly.

During my early 20's, I struggled with a lot of fatigue, especially after lunchtime. I turned to coffee and caffeine to get through the day. I never worked full-time and would always wonder how other co-workers could work full-time, have a full weekend of activity, and be back at work on Monday. Some of my days off of work were spent trying to recover from working just a few days in a row. I always blew it off, saying I did a lot of other things at home like having a large garden, canning lots of vegetables, cooking, etc.

July 5th 2011, my husband developed severe sinus drainage, ear pressure, joint pain, fatigue, etc. He had been having fun with firecrackers on the 4th of July, so we thought with the timing that all these symptoms may just have been due to the loud noise.

After these symptoms continued for a few months, he finally went to the doctor and was given a round of antibiotics and antihistamines, none of which did anything for his symptoms. The sinus symptoms finally subsided a bit, but he was left with chronic pain and tightness in his shoulders and neck, and a squeezing pressure in his head. The next few years anytime he would get an illness or cold, the sinus symptoms would flare up. We decided to try a more natural approach using chiropractic and a massage therapist who performed myofascial release. We could never find anything that truly worked for him. Now, many years later, we believe these were his first symptoms of Lyme. He never had a tick bite or rash that we could identify.

That same fall of 2011, I developed severe neck and shoulder pain as well. At the time I thought it was related to how much canning and vegetable processing I was doing. I now look back and believe that these were symptoms of a Lyme infection for me as well.

In 2013 after a very stressful event in our lives, I developed Iritis in one of my eyes. Iritis is an auto-immune inflammation of the iris in the eye. It felt like I had knives stabbing the back of my eyeball every time my iris would dilate or constrict as it naturally does when exposed to bright light or when focusing in on something close up. This process happens thousands of times per day. I didn't know why this had happened, but was happy when it was gone with the use of many eye drops.

My eyelid also developed a twitch, so the eye doctor recommended trying eye drops for dry eyes. The twitching would last for a few days and then go away so I wasn't too concerned.

Unfortunately I developed iritis again within 6 months of the first occurrence. This time the eye doctor recommended getting tested for other autoimmune conditions. Iritis is common if a person has something like Rheumatoid Arthritis, Ankylosing Spondylitis, MS, etc. I decided not to go through with testing since I didn't have any joint pain or other symptoms of an autoimmune disease and I had already decided I would not take pharmaceutical medications for an autoimmune condition.

Following this second bout of Iritis I was fairly concerned that I would continue to develop Iritis. For treatment, I was given steroid eye drops. I did some reading about steroid eye drops and after about 700 doses steroid induced cataracts can develop. I was 27 years old at the time and even though I took care of patients who have cataract surgeries, and know it is a simple procedure, I did not want to have cataract surgery so young.

Every month following that, with monthly hormonal changes, I would feel the pain of the Iritis coming back. I resorted to taking a few ibuprofen when I would feel the pain, and thankfully never developed full blown Iritis again. I always felt like there had to be something that had caused the Iritis.

June 7th, 2014 - The day that changed my life. I found a tiny deer tick on my finger by my wedding ring.

At this point I did not know anything about Lyme disease except that most people diagnosed were very sick. I researched a few things, but tried not to worry about it.

A week later, I woke up and my knee joints were sore and achy. By 10 days after the tick bite, I could hardly walk 1000feet without my knees feeling incredibly sore and my leg muscles incredibly weak. I felt I was going to collapse. I had many flu like symptoms and felt like my body was "fighting something".

I was unable to get an appointment with a Lyme literate doctor in the area and finally went to see an Internal Medicine doctor. This doctor was less than helpful and made me feel like I was crazy. This doctor suggested that we do Rheumatoid Arthritis testing instead, which I refused. I had never had joint pain like this before in my life and then to have it about a week after a tick bite? It was too much of a coincidence for it not to be an infection. I finally convinced this doctor to give me 10 days of Doxycycline. Interesting note - Doxycycline is easily prescribed for months to years for patients with acne, but it was like pulling teeth to have it prescribed for a possible Lyme infection!

Within 2 days of taking the antibiotic, the joint pain in my knees was about 75% better. I did have a lot of lymph node swelling and detox symptoms while on the antibiotic. Despite my ELISA test coming back negative, I suspected that I had a Lyme infection.

The 10 days of Doxycycline was not enough to

eradicate the Lyme infection but the doctor would not give me more. I finally found a natural option which used homeopathics to support my own immune system in fighting the infection.

While I was on a 2 month course of this therapy, the joint pain went away, the symptoms of Iritis went away, the eye lid twitching went away. It was amazing! Later, when more testing came back it appeared that I had a chronic Lyme infection as well as this recent tick bite that had caused the acute infection.

While I was going through all of this, I would tell my husband my symptoms, and he would say "welcome to my life the last few years". I started to wonder if he also had a Lyme infection. All of his tests came back looking like he did. So he started on the homeopathics as well.

We were on the right track using the homeopathics to allow the immune system to fight the infection itself, and were led to believe that one round was enough. Unfortunately, the doctor assisting us with the homeopathics didn't do further testing to truly make sure the Lyme infection was gone. There are no lab tests that can be used for this which I will discuss later on.

Since we were led to believe Lyme was behind us, the next months we found a local naturopath to help us work on what we thought was the damage that years of Lyme had caused, adrenals, thyroid, liver congestion, toxins in the body, etc.

This was challenging and it felt like we were always chasing "this" symptom or trying to get to the root of "that" problem, and it would change with every appointment. We finally discovered after many months of frustration and continuing to feel worse, that the underlying cause was still an ongoing Lyme infection.

After many years and countless dollars spent on trying just about EVERYTHING, we finally found a doctor out of state that used some alternative testing methods to be able to clearly monitor how long therapy needed to continue. Along with a Lyme infection for me, he found numerous other infections, some of them considered to be co-infections that frequently 'travel' along with Lyme. Since both my husband and I had these chronic infections for many years, it wasn't an easy or quick road back to health, but truly life changing to finally find a practitioner who had the answers and who had been in our shoes. Lyme is a 'smart' bug that shuts down the immune system. It wears the body down to the point that my husband especially was very sick. At my low point, I was barely able to work 2 days per week but now I am thriving and feeling better than I ever remember feeling! We are on the path to healing and it is my hope and prayer that this book can be useful in explaining some of the confusion surrounding Lyme.

Chapter 1: Lyme Disease - The Fastest Growing Infection of Modern Time

Borrelia Burgdorferi....Say what? Borrelia is the bacteria that causes Lyme disease. It is a spirochete shaped bacteria that burrows into tissues and organs, is very smart and when threatened, can change form into cysts. These cysts can stay dormant until they are no longer threatened by the immune system or antibiotics/herbs. At that time, the cysts can "hatch" out and cause further infection. Borrelia prefers to move through the connective tissue of the body, not the blood. To complete its lifecycle, Borrelia needs manganese and magnesium, which are found in the connective tissues, not the blood.

Borrelia spirochetes are able to pass into the brain through the blood brain barrier and there are some who believe that this can sometimes happen within the first 24 hours of infection. The fact that Borrelia hides in tissue and not blood makes it hard to detect using standard blood testing.

There are many theories of where Lyme came from, and why it is causing such a spread of infection. That isn't the point of this book and there are many other books that explore that subject. I am writing this book to be able to give others a reference on a subject that has taken me many years of research to understand. If you are new to Lyme disease, you have most likely found a vast array of confusing and contradictory information on the internet, books and from your doctor. Information from the CDC telling you one thing, information from other sources telling you something completely different and still other Lyme message boards with other information. When I first had my tick bite, my head was spinning from all of the very different information that I found within just the first few hours of searching. I want this book to hopefully clarify some of these contradictions for others.

Borrelia is considered to be a cousin to Syphillis, and has been called the 'great imitator' because of its ability to cause so many symptoms related to so many diseases. The symptoms caused by it can mimic symptoms from 80 different diseases. EVERYONE has different symptoms associated with a Borrelia infection, no two people are the same in how symptoms manifest. Therefore, it is very difficult to diagnose and many times the real infection goes undiagnosed, while the person is incorrectly diagnosed with various conditions depending on what symptoms they may have.
Borrelia usually does not travel alone. There are numerous co-infections that can come along with it. Babesia, Bartonella, Ehrlichia, Mycoplasma, Cytomegalovirus, Rickettsia, Powassan, etc. These cause a whole host of other symptoms.

The symptoms of Lyme disease vary greatly from person to person. My personal symptoms were:
-Muscle pain

-Migrating joint pain, bilateral knee pain, small joint pain in my fingers, TMJ pain
-Iritis (Autoimmune inflammation of the iris of the eye)
-Fatigue
-Short-term memory problems and significant brain fog
-Mixing up words or not being able to think of the word that I wanted to say
-Fatigue
-Eyelid twitching
-Hormone imbalance

Some of the other symptoms associated with Lyme disease:
-Bull's eye rash
-High fever, chills or sweating
-Flu-like symptoms
-Headaches
-Muscle and joint pain
-Bell's palsy
-Confusion, getting lost or becoming disoriented
-Feeling lightheaded
-Depression and mood swings
-Sleep disturbances
-Fatigue
-Visual problems – floaters, blurriness, light sensitivity
-Eye pressure
-Stiff or sore back or joints
-Neck pain, stiffness, creaks or cracks

-Shooting pains, numbness, burning, tingling or stabbing sensations
-Heart palpitations or chest pain
-Coughing or feeling short of breath
-Ringing in ears or sudden hearing loss
-Vertigo, poor balance, or motion sickness
-Tremors
-Swollen glands
-Weight loss or gain
-Irregular menstrual periods
-Bladder dysfunction or irritability
-Abdominal pain or upset stomach
-Sensation of electrical shocks in the head or down the spine
-Abnormal heart rhythm, Atrial Fibrilation

Some incorrect diagnoses that are associated when Lyme disease is the underlying cause.
-Alzheimers
-Multiple sclerosis
-Rheumatoid Arthritis
-Lupus
-ALS
-Chronic fatigue
-Fibromyalgia
-Parkinson's
-Lou Gehrig's disease

As mentioned earlier, every individual has different symptoms. Some may have severe symptoms and end up in the hospital. Others may have almost no symptoms or very minor symptoms. And still others, suffer with chronic, unexplained symptoms and are diagnosed with autoimmune diseases or other degenerative diseases.

Lyme is classified by how long the person has had the disease, where it has spread throughout the body, and what other body systems are affected and showing symptoms.

Early Localized Lyme

When Lyme is in the acute stage (recent infection or known recent tick bite), it is most easily treated with a course of antibiotics. The antibiotic needs to be started as soon as possible, while the infection is still in the blood stream and able to be killed by the antibiotic. Will the antibiotic take care of the Lyme infection for every person? Quite possibly, but my conclusion along with many other doctors is that it may need to be followed up by other therapy.

When there is a known tick bite, less than 50% of people develop the classic Bull's eye rash associated with Lyme disease. Many times there is the appearance of a rash, but it does not manifest as a bull's eye. Other times, people don't remember seeing a rash at all. I never had a rash, despite knowing that I had a tick bite and developing knee pain within 1 week of the bite.

With the rash, many times there are flu-like

symptoms, fevers, muscle soreness, headaches.
Even if there is no rash, but flu-like symptoms appear after a known tick bite, or after outdoor activities, it is important to take measures to address the possible Lyme infection.

Sometimes people may experience a brief flu-like illness, minor joint pain, etc. Then all the symptoms subside and the person believes that all is well. In reality, the Borrelia is lying dormant in the body for a time that the immune system becomes stressed, is compromised, and then starts attacking the body.

Early Disseminated Lyme

This stage of Lyme happens when the Borrelia bacteria has spread outside of the bloodstream and is affecting other parts of the body. Borrelia loves the connective tissues so symptoms like muscle, joint, and tendon pain appear. These pains often migrate around the body. Borrelia may also start to affect the heart, causing palpitations and it may start to affect the neurological system which may cause Bell's palsy, cranial nerve issues, meningitis, stiff neck, sensitivity to light, headaches, fatigue, dizziness, burning or shooting pains, etc. Other cognitive changes that can be seen are memory loss, difficulty concentrating or focusing, "brain fog". Some of the psychological symptoms can include irritability, obsessive compulsive traits, and severe anxiety.

Chronic Lyme Disease

When Lyme has disseminated into the body and gone untreated for months to years, it is considered to be chronic Lyme. Some doctors may call this Post Treatment Lyme Disease. The Infections Diseases Society of America (IDSA) denies that chronic Lyme disease exists. This, along with poor methods of lab testing make a Lyme diagnosis difficult to obtain from a conventional doctor, despite the fact a person may have so many symptoms. Many doctors unfortunately believe that Lyme is difficult to catch, and easy to treat. Quite the contrary when you start to talk with people whose lives have been impacted by chronic Lyme.

ILADS (International Lyme and Associated Diseases Society) has guidelines for persistent Lyme disease
-symptoms that continue despite 30 days of treatment
-recurrent Lyme disease – the patient relapsing in the absence of another tick bite or rash
-refractory Lyme disease – a patient responding poorly to antibiotic therapy.

In the case of Chronic Lyme Disease, my opinion is that antibiotics are less effective because the Borrelia spirochetes enter into the connective tissue, organs, brain, and other places of the body that are less vascular. Antibiotics can kill spirochetes in the blood, but aren't effective against spirochetes in the tissues, organs, brain, etc. In addition to antibiotics not being very effective, when the Borrelia spirochetes feel like they are being attacked, they form into cysts. These cysts are able to convert back into spirochete form when they feel they are no longer being threatened and cause a worsening of infection. Antibiotics are not capable of killing the cyst form of Borrelia.

Autoimmunity related to Lyme

When Borrelia is present in the body, the immune system may have been activated to look for 'invaders'. However, as soon as the Borrelia spirochete feels threatened, it changes form and the immune system can't find the 'invader' so it begins to attack different tissues in the body. This is where many of the autoimmune symptoms related to a Lyme infection originate.

Prevalence of Lyme

According to the CDC's website. "Each year, approximately 30,000 cases of Lyme disease are reported to CDC by state health departments and the District of Columbia. However, this number does not reflect every case of Lyme disease that is diagnosed in the United States every year."
Many researchers estimate that the actual number of

Lyme cases each year in the United States is at least 10 fold higher than the number reported to the CDC.

Even that number is thought to be lower than the actual number of cases per year, given the difficulty in testing and the large range of Borrelial species.

As we will discuss in Chapter 2, the current testing for Lyme and co-infections is ineffective. I believe that many symptoms are not recognized by doctors as being related to an underlying infection. Conventional medicine focuses more on treating symptoms and not as much or at all on identifying the root cause of why the symptoms are manifesting. Often arthritis is blamed on old age, joint pain blamed on over work, fatigue and exhaustion blamed on being too busy and stressed, etc. What if there are truly chronic infections underlying and causing these symptoms?

Chapter 2: Transmission Routes and Why Conventional Testing is Not Reliable

When someone mentions Lyme disease, we all think of a deer tick bite and bulls eye rash. Yet, there are many other ways for Lyme disease to be transmitted. Yes, the deer tick bite is often associated with someone developing symptoms of Lyme and correctly so. But, it is estimated that only about 1/3rd of those infected with Lyme will actually display a bulls eye rash.

For myself, when I discovered a deer tick bite several years ago, I never developed a bulls eye rash.

Less than 50% of people with Lyme disease recall being bitten by a tick. It's possible and probable that mosquitos, deer flies, horse flies and spiders are also able to transmit Borrelia spirochetes and other co-infections to humans and animals.

Some researchers and doctors believe that not everyone exposed to Borrelia will experience symptoms or develop a Lyme infection. I believe it depends on the individual's immune system and how well the immune system is functioning. What other things like heavy metals, toxicity, poor nutrition, and other infections might be impairing healthy immune function? Lyme is opportunistic. If there is a breakdown, the Lyme infection can take over when the immune system isn't able to defend against it.

Another transmission route that is extremely important to be aware of is sexual transmission. This could be the way both my husband and I became infected.
Even though it may not be the most comfortable topic to discuss, it is very important to be aware of this route of transmission. There have been many studies done where partners have been tested and show the exact strains of Lyme disease (there are many different strains). How is that possible besides sexual transmission? It is important to test the partner of the patient with Lyme and to use safe sex practices.

Unfortunately, despite many other studies, the CDC still claims that Lyme disease is not spread from person to person through sexual contact or saliva. [6]
Another important mode of transmission to be aware of is congenital transmission. Transmission from a mother to her child during pregnancy. Sometimes entire families are infected. If you have a suspected Lyme infection, get tested prior to becoming pregnant if possible. A Borrelia infection in the mother can cause pregnancy loss or birth defects. Is

every baby with an infected mother born with a Lyme infection? No, but they may likely be born with the infection. If the infection is present in the baby, is Lyme going to manifest itself in the newborn immediately? Not necessarily, it depends on what other infections or immune system problems might be present. Lyme is a very smart bacteria and will often 'lie in wait' and then when the immune system becomes compromised, start to manifest itself.

There have been some newer studies done that show Borrelia spirochetes can be present in saliva, urine, tears and breast milk.

Testing

Testing is a difficult topic to discuss. You would think that modern, conventional medicine would have a test that would readily discover this infection that is challenging so many people. Sadly, most lab testing methods are extremely inaccurate.

Two tiered testing

In the US, we have something called two tiered testing. This means that when you go to your doctor's office, they will do a blood draw. The lab will initially run an ELISA test, and if that comes back positive, will then run a Western Blot test.

There have been advances in the last several years and some doctors will now order the Western Blot first and skip the ELISA test.

ELISA - enzyme-linked immunosorbent assay. This test uses blood or spinal fluid to test for the presence of anti-bodies to Borrelia bacteria. Unfortunately, the ELISA test has proven that it is not all that effective in the diagnosis of Lyme disease. Generally, 40% of people that have the bull's eye rash, indicating exposure to Lyme disease will test negative for Lyme using the ELISA test. The body won't produce the antibodies needed for detection with ELISA until 2-4 weeks after infection!

The Western Blot test is not much more effective than the ELISA test in diagnosing Lyme. The Western Blot test was originally designed to be a surveillance test, not a diagnostic test. Having a Western Blot done early on in a suspected Lyme exposure, is not very reliable. It takes about 4-6 weeks for the body to produce antibodies that can be recognized by the Western Blot. Also, unfortunately, years ago the CDC eliminated the use of 31kd and 34kd bands in this test even though these bands were the ones proven to be most indicative of Lyme exposure. It is believed that these bands were removed when the Lyme vaccine was trialed in the 1990's, because they didn't want to cause confusion in someone who had received the Lyme vaccine. If a person was to get the vaccine, the 31kd and 34kd bands would turn positive. The Lyme vaccine was a horrible failure, giving 1/10th to 1/3rd of those who had received it symptoms of Lyme disease or the actual disease. It was removed from use in 2002.

To be considered CDC positive for Lyme disease the following must apply. "It was recommended that an IgM immunoblot be considered positive if two of the following three bands are present: 24 kDa (OspC) *, 39 kDa (BmpA), and 41 kDa (Fla) (1). It was further recommended that an that IgG immunoblot be considered positive if five of the following 10 bands are present: 18 kDa, 21 kDa (OspC) *, 28 kDa, 30 kDa, 39 kDa (BmpA), 41 kDa (Fla), 45 kDa, 58 kDa (not GroEL), 66 kDa, and 93 kDa (2)."

The Western Blot from Igenex is considered to give a more conclusive result. It is an expanded Western Blot test that looks for more bands that are indicative of a Lyme infection. Most Lyme Literate MDs or other practitioners that are well versed in Lyme disease believe that just one positive band is significant. Igenex also does co-infection testing. Most likely, this lab test will not be covered by insurance as they are classified as experimental and the test is not FDA approved.

When Lyme goes undetected and untreated for a period of time, it becomes chronic. It's a very smart bug as it down-regulates the immune system, causing it to not function properly. By the time most people start to suspect they have a chronic Lyme infection due to their symptoms, the body is already quite sick. When a person is already quite sick with Lyme, the immune system is not strong enough to show the antibodies in the blood. Basically, you have to be well enough to actually be fighting the infection for it to show up on a Western Blot test. You would think the more positive bands on a test, the worse the patient's infection would be. The opposite may be true as Lyme disease shuts down the immune system. At times the people who are the sickest, have the fewest or no bands that are positive. Even though they have a less positive result, that doesn't mean that they are less sick!

Because of all of the above, Lyme disease, especially Chronic Lyme disease is difficult to diagnose. The ELISA and Western Blot tests only show exposure and antibodies to Borrelia, not if there is an active infection.

In the last few years, there is a new test called the iSpot Lyme test that is thought to be more accurate for testing. The iSpot Lyme test uses the T-cell part of the immune system which generally mounts a measurable response to a pathogen like Borrelia within 2 weeks of infection versus the Western Blot's 4-6 weeks after infection.

Dr Myerowitz, D.C., Dilp. Ac. (NCCAOM), Lac., F.I.C.C., DABCA, BCIM has his "22 reasons for having a negative Lyme diagnosis based on bloodwork.

1. You were recently infected and tested before your body produced Lyme antibodies.
2. You took antibiotics before testing, which co-opted an antibody response.
3. You were already on long-term antibiotics for another illness.
4. Not enough "free" Lyme antibodies were detectable in your blood because they were all doing their job binding to the Lyme bacteria.
5. Lyme spirochetes were protected and hiding inside a biofilm colony
6. Spirochetes were burrowed deep inside your body (ie, cartilage, fibroblasts, neurons, etc.).
7. Only small blebs were in your body, no whole bacteria, which are needed for the PCR (Polymerase Chain Reaction) based tests.
8. There are no free Spirochetes in the body fluid on day of test.
9. Genetic heterogeneity – there are at least 300 strains of Lyme, 100 in the U.S. You might be infected by a strain of Borrelia that the test doesn't recognize.

10. Antigen variability – Borrelia can change its outer surface protein to suit its environment so the test will detect a "non-Lyme specific" antibody.
11. Spirochetes are in dormancy phase (L-form) with no cell walls, so there is nothing for the immune system to attack with antibodies.
12. Lyme's surface antigens can change body temperature
13. You have an immune deficiency.
14. You have had recent anti-inflammatory treatment which suppresses the immune system.
15. Co-infection with Babesia (protozoa) which causes immune suppression.
16. Down-regulation of your immune system by your body's own cytokines.
17. Lab error or poor technical capability/training to detect Lyme disease.
18. You might have late stage Lyme. Lab tests are not standardized for detecting late stage Lyme disease.
19. The lab tests might only have been approved for investigational use
20. Lack of adequate reference points for the test (most tests only use a few genetic strains as reference).
21. The revised Western Blot Criteria fails to include important Antibody Bands.

22.Centers for Disease Control testing criteria is designed for epidemiological study, not clinical diagnostics."

(Reprinted with permission)

Alternative Types of Testing

Through personal experience and meeting some amazing practitioners, we have found better success with alternative types of testing. We found that while there are some blood tests that can tell you that you may have had an exposure to Lyme disease, there is no lab test that can reliably tell if the therapy you are doing is actually working. From a lab test there was no way to tell if the infection was still present, active, if the therapy was working, or if you had cleared the infection and it was no longer disrupting the body.

This was quite frustrating. How do you know how long to continue on the therapy you are doing? How do you know if what you are doing is actually working? How do you know if your immune system has become strong enough that Lyme is not constantly disrupting the body?

Finally, in answer to these questions, we found a doctor who uses an electrodermal screening device. This device pulses tiny electrical currents into the body and judges the body's response to those specific frequencies. Highly specialized computer software runs this device and is used to detect imbalances in the body, bacteria, viruses, toxins, vitamin and mineral deficiencies, etc. With this method these imbalances can be detected long before blood work would show anything or the person would start showing symptoms. Natural medicine believes that the body is designed to heal, it just needs the interference (toxins, heavy metals, infections, etc.) removed and also the correct nutrients and minerals to be available. By correcting these imbalances, the body can start to heal itself. This is the whole principle of using homeopathy to heal from chronic infections. It gives the body the information it needs so the body's own immune system can systematically eliminate and fight the Lyme or other chronic infection.

A little background on electrodermal screening, as it seems foreign at first. It has been used by mainstream medicine in Russia and Europe for many years. There are reports that NASA astronauts use electrodermal screening while in space to identify imbalances in the body before disease symptoms manifest.

This is a primary method of testing I use at my office to determine what is causing imbalances in the body. I can then use other methods of testing to find the remedies that balance the body so that it can start to heal.

At the risk of sounding like I'm into 'new age' energy, I need to talk about the energy of the body. It sounded strange and different to me at first, but then I researched it more in depth. Our bodies have energy driving all of our functions; our heart uses electrical impulses to beat. Conventional medicine acknowledges that an EKG of the heart measures the electrical conduction of the heart. We have energy all throughout our bodies and this energy drives all of the normal functions of the body. The brain sends nerve impulses/energy to the fingers causing them to move, etc.

This leads into muscle testing, which also sounded strange to me at first. I've been able to see firsthand the amazing information that this can gather from the body. Learning how to muscle test has helped me personally and is another important method of testing I use at my practice. It helps to pinpoint the dysfunction and find the root cause. With this method I can then also find solutions that help to balance the body so it can truly heal.

Muscle testing is used to identify various imbalances in the body. This is done using the strength of the muscle as an extension of the nervous system. Every bacteria, virus, toxin, herb, nutrient, or living thing has a unique frequency. Using vials with these unique frequencies contained in them, the practitioner can determine what frequencies are disrupting the body. The practitioner can place these vials up against the body and assess the strength of the muscle versus when the vial was not placed up against the body. When the vials/frequencies that are challenging the body are discovered, there is a clear response from the body. The disrupting frequency in such close proximity overwhelms the brain and nervous system and causes a significant weakening in the muscle.

The practitioner doing the muscle testing can also use muscle testing to assess the organs and lymphatic drainage of the body. This is done by the tester placing his/her hand over various organs and assessing muscle strength. When there is a stressed organ in the body, the small amount of additional stress caused on that organ by the tester placing his/her hand over that area, again causes a significant weakening in the muscle. This weakening happens because the brain and nervous system became stressed and over-loaded. The body can no longer handle the added stress and maintain a strong muscle.

By finding these imbalances using "problem" vials, the practitioner then finds "solutions". A herb, food, mineral, homeopathic, or nutritional supplement that balance out the body. When the practitioner holds both the "problems" and correct "solutions" up to the body, now the body is balanced and the muscle is able to stay strong!

Using muscle testing, the practitioner is able to develop a specific protocol for each client. No body is the same, everyone is unique as are their nutritional needs. Muscle testing also allows the body to prioritize what is most important to deal with presently and not forcing the body to do something that it is not ready to do. This helps to minimize detox reactions though symptoms can still occur as they are part of the healing process of the body.

My personal experience with both electrodermal screening and muscle testing has been incredible.

Chapter 3: Coinfections

Borrelia does not travel alone. We need to take into consideration that ticks and other insects carry many different bacteria, viruses, and parasites.

Why is this important? Many people go through treatment for Lyme disease, but if the other co-infections are present and not dealt with also, symptoms may remain.

If the immune system is suppressed from numerous infections by bacteria, viruses, or parasites, a new infection can occur more easily if there is exposure. In these cases the symptoms are likely to be more severe.

Babesia

Babesia is thought to infect nearly 100% of those infected with Borrelia (Lyme).

It is a parasitic infection that lives inside the red blood cells.

Babesia symptoms can be varied, some are:
- Severe headaches
- Drenching night sweats and sometimes day sweats (some menopausal women think that they are having hot flashes, make sure to check for infection with Babesia)

- Air hunger, shortness of breath
- Sighing
- Bell's palsy
- Dizziness, light-headedness
- Flushing
- Flare-ups every 4-6 days
- Neurological symptoms
- Feeling of spaciness, wooziness, and impending doom
- GI issues, nausea, intestinal discomfort, bloating after eating
- Hormone imbalance

Bartonella

Bartonella has been known as "Cat Scratch Fever". It is a bacteria.

Symptoms are varied and include:

- Sharp pains in the soles of the feet (symptoms similar to neuropathy or plantar fasciitis)
- Headaches or Migraines
- Sensations of something crawling under the skin
- Digestive issues such as gastritis, abdominal pain, IBD
- Muscle twitches, and tremor related to Central Nervous System irritability
- Anxiety, mood swings, antisocial behavior, OCD
- Swollen lymph nodes

- Stretch marks in new places that can be white or red/purple in color
- Rapid heart rate

Ehrlichia

Ehrlichia is a form of rickettsiales bacteria.
Some of the symptoms include:

- Muscle pain (differing from the joint pain associated with Lyme)
- Pain in the tendons
- Neurological problems such as seizure disorders and shooting pains
- Sharp, knife-like headaches that are often behind the eyes
- Low White Blood Cell count with elevated liver enzymes
- Right upper quadrant pain in abdomen

Mycoplasma

Mycoplasma are a type of bacteria that lack a cell wall. They are the smallest and simplest organism known. Mycoplasma are the microorganisms associated with Gulf War Illness.
Some of the symptoms associated with Mycoplasma infection include:

- Intermittent fevers
- Night sweats
- Memory loss

- Fatigue
- Visual disturbances
- Abnormal blood pressure
- Gastrointestinal problems, nausea, bloating, diarrhea
- Walking pneumonia
- Slowly worsening cough that lasts for weeks to months

These are only a few of the co-infections that are most commonly present along with a Lyme infection. There can also be viral infections, bacteria infections as well as parasite infections.

It is important to understand the complexity of Lyme and these possible co-infections. Sometimes, they need to be dealt with individually, and sometimes after the body has dealt with the "priority" infection(s), the immune system is then able to handle some of the lesser challenges on its own.

Chapter 4: Why "Just Killing the Bugs" using Antibiotics isn't the Answer

Acute Lyme: Antibiotic vs. Homeopathy

When Lyme is in the acute stage (recent infection or known recent tick bite), it is most easily treatable with a course of antibiotics. The antibiotic needs to be started as soon as possible, while the infection is still in the blood stream and able to be killed by the antibiotic. Will the antibiotic take care of the Lyme infection for every person? Quite possibly, but it may need to be followed up by other therapy or at least further testing.

What about co-infections, like Babesia that are parasites and are not "killed" by antibiotics? Given the limitations of standard blood testing that we discussed earlier, I personally would recommend seeking further testing. The earlier the problem is found, the easier it will be to solve.

Chronic Lyme

So, you were fortunate enough to get a Lyme diagnosis by a conventional doctor, but you've had these horrible symptoms and have been sick for many years. Or you look at the clinical signs and symptoms that you've had for many years and they match up with many of the symptoms of Lyme disease. Either way, you have chronic Lyme, not acute. If you are seeing a Lyme Literate MD he/she most likely will give you a treatment plan that may consist of months to years of antibiotics, perhaps pulsed with anti-fungals, or anti-parasitic medications depending on what co-infections were also found. Unfortunately, most of these doctors talk little or nothing about repairing and rebuilding the immune system along with "killing the bugs".

I don't believe this is the answer for Chronic Lyme. By this time, Borrelia has become a chronic infection. It has invaded the connective tissue, the joints, the brain, organs, the extracellular matrix (space between the cells), etc. Antibiotics or antibiotic type herbs work best when there is an acute infection in the blood or vascular tissues. Connective tissue isn't very vascular, meaning the antibiotics can't get to the bacteria very well or attack it. Even when the bacteria is in more vascular places, it can be quite difficult to eradicate. The Borrelia bacteria is called a 'smart' bug, and has between 7 and 23 plasmids that are able to make the bacteria change form into dormant cysts. To put this into perspective, a common staph bacteria that causes a staph infection contains only 3 plasmids, making it much easier to eradicate using antibiotics. It can't change form as quickly or resist antibiotics as well as Borrelia. There are studies showing that within minutes of exposure to antibiotics, Borrelia can change into cyst form. This drives the infection deeper into the body, and antibiotics are not effective against the cyst form of Borrelia. A good example is Doxycycline. It will reduce the spirochete form by approximately 90%, but will immediately double the number of cyst forms. I believe that the same thing happens when taking herbal "killers".

I know many who have tried the antibiotic or herbal "killer" route of treatment for chronic Lyme. They have been on antibiotics many years, and may feel better while taking the antibiotics. But, as soon as they stop them, a few weeks or months later, the Lyme symptoms return. This is most likely because the antibiotics or herbals have turned the Borrelia into cyst form. As soon as the coast is clear, the cysts 'hatch' and cause another Borrelia infection that needs to be dealt with yet again.

The other problem antibiotics cause is down-regulation of the immune system. This is most likely the reason people feel better while taking the antibiotics. The immune system is suppressed and most symptoms are also suppressed. Most symptoms related to the Lyme infection are thought to come from the immune system trying to fight the infection.

Also, antibiotics wreak havoc in the gut. One short 10 day course of antibiotics has been shown to wipe out 1/3 of the good bacteria in the gut! What happens when you take months to years of antibiotics? Sometimes even combinations of several different antibiotics! We need the good bacteria in our gut for our immune system to function well, to assist us with digestion, and to help keep pathogenic or bad bacteria under control (i.e. Candida). Studies show that over 70% of our immune system is located in our gut in the gut-associated lymphoid tissue (GALT) and the mucosal-associated lymphoid tissue (MALT). There is also a connection between the gut and the brain. The gut is responsible for making many different hormones and neurotransmitters, like dopamine, serotonin, etc. These are all very important for healthy mood and brain function.

Antibiotics are full of synthetic chemicals that the body must process or store away if unable to process. Many are made from Petroleum products. Antibiotics can cause liver and kidney damage. While undergoing treatment, doctors will monitor liver and kidney function every month. When Lyme disease is present, there is most likely some liver dysfunction already, so compounding the problem by taking toxic pharmaceuticals can make the problem worse.

It's important to look at why Lyme occurred in the first place. Not everyone exposed to Borrelia bacteria will develop symptoms of Lyme disease. There is a correlation between a low functioning immune system and symptoms. We need to look for the underlying causes of a low functioning immune system such as other chronic infections, leaky gut, heavy metals, toxicity, stress, etc. If these underlying causes are not dealt with, the Lyme infection and other chronic infections will keep coming back. If you are using something like antibiotics that drive the Borrelia infection into cyst form, and never completely kill the entire infection, how can you ever expect to be well when the medications are causing low immune function and other dysfunction in the body?

What if we took a different approach than just "killing the bugs"? Perhaps an approach that looks at the entire body, and not just covering symptoms. Assessing organ dysfunction, looking for heavy metals, toxicity, leaky gut, emotional stress, etc., and recognizing that the body is designed to heal. We need to remove the interference, the toxicity, give the body the right information and nutrients needed and the body will heal. Our bodies show extreme intelligence in design and are not the product of a slow evolutionary process. Our immune systems, when not compromised by the toxic world around us are designed to protect us from these challenges. How can we support our bodies and correct the damage that has been done. I believe God is our Creator and our Great Physician, He can heal our bodies in any way He chooses, but I also believe that He gave us knowledge and tools to use, the ability to study, research and learn.

So, let's work to "Lyme proof your immune system"!

Chapter 5: Using Homeopathy to Deal with Chronic Infections

We've already discussed how antibiotic and herbal protocols are not very effective when dealing with a Lyme infection or other chronic infection. When a Lyme infection becomes chronic, it can cause autoimmunity and other related issues. The immune system has been stimulated to "kill the bugs", but can't find them because of how "smart" a bug Lyme is in hiding from the immune system. If the immune system then starts to attack other parts of the body, stimulating the immune system with various herbs that have powerful immune stimulation properties, only causes more autoimmunity in the body, making symptoms worse. This is where homeopathy comes in as the ideal way of helping the body to deal with the infection(s).

We have to get past the "kill the bugs" mentality. Homeopathy works in a completely different way. It works with instead of against your immune system.

What is homeopathy? Homeopathy was created by Samuel Hahnemann in the 1790's, and is based on his discovery that "like can cure like". This means that a substance given to a healthy person would cause symptoms, but given to a sick person, would help alleviate symptoms and allow the body to heal.

A good example of this is the herb nux vomica. In a healthy person, high doses would cause nausea. Dilute doses given to a person with nausea, alleviate the symptom of nausea. Homeopathics are made by taking a substance and diluting it with alcohol or distilled water. Continuing this dilution until there is hardly any of the original substance, but the energetic frequencies of the herb or various other substance remain within the solution. Hahnemann was surprised to find that the more dilute the solution was, the faster and more effective it was.

Homeopathy was a very common practice in the United States in the 1800s and early 1900s. The practice was even taught in Medical colleges. When antibiotics and pharmaceuticals became popular in the 1930's and 1940's, the use of homeopathy to help the body heal started to decrease in the US.

In the last number of years, homeopathy has been increasing in popularity, especially with people seeking alternative therapies, as we see the incidence of chronic disease skyrocketing and antibiotic resistance growing.

Dr Cahis, a Spanish homeopath, developed serial remedies in 1911. This involved taking a different dilution of a specific homeopathic each day or every few days. He found this to be an effective means of dealing with various infections.

There is a homeopathic company that has taken this concept and has developed a line of serial remedies for many chronic infections. This is what I have used personally with great success and what I recommend to my clients. The reason this homeopathic line is so effective is that they are made from a "mother tincture". For example, to make a Borrelia serial remedy, they take <u>inactivated</u> Borrelia bacteria and make a mother tincture. Then they dilute to the specific dilution needed. This leaves a tiny bit of the Borrelia DNA in the homeopathic solution. This is what the body needs to truly heal. It gives the immune system the information it needs to find and fight the infection(s).

And no, you cannot get a Borrelia infection from taking Borrelia homeopathics. They use inactivated (i.e. killed) substances in the making of all homeopathics.

This company's serial remedies are considered to be some of the top natural remedies for dealing with Lyme and other co-infection symptoms. Their products are only available through healthcare practitioners and should only be used under the direction of an experienced practitioner.

Serial Remedies

So how do serial remedies work? The homeopathics are taken every third day for 2 months or as directed by your practitioner. The first month series up-regulates the immune system to fight the infection, and the second month down-regulates the immune system, turning off the antibody response so that the immune system is not constantly looking for something to fight.

When the two months are completed, testing is done to see if the body is ready to go on to the next phase of dealing with the infection. It is quite common, especially with chronic Lyme to repeat this first round of serial remedies multiple times before the body is ready to move on. When ready, the next phase can last between 10 and 20 weeks. By taking higher dilutions of homeopathics once or twice per week as directed, the body finishes flushing out the infection. This next phase also provides an amount of passive immunity to the infection that was just fought (this has been noted clinically, but hasn't been proven through lab testing). This therapy is similar to the principle of vaccination, except without all of the toxic ingredients and contaminants that are contained in vaccines….another subject for another time.

How do you feel during this? It is important to remember that symptoms are indications that the body is fighting (i.e. healing). It is important to work with an experienced practitioner to determine what your body needs and what it is ready for. This minimizes detox or clearing reactions. Everyone is different with how they feel. Most can continue to go about their normal routines, others are fairly sick during this time. As your immune system fights these infections, toxins are released. Some of the ill feelings, herxheimer reactions, or clearing reactions can be due to the toxins being released and the detoxification system of the body getting overwhelmed. This is why it is important to work with an experienced practitioner during this time as they can suggest natural and homeopathic products to assist the body with this detoxification process. Although no one wants to feel unwell, symptoms after beginning this process can be a good thing. It is proof that you are on the right track and your immune system is fighting.

Specific organ support may be needed during this time as often the liver and kidneys become overwhelmed. There are many herbal and homeopathic support products that are helpful with this.

Also, some need additional Lymphatic Support. The lymphatic system is a very important part of the circulation and immune system and helps to rid the body of toxins. I typically use homeopathics or a liposomal Vitamin C to support the lymphatic system. The homeopathics help to open up the drainage pathways so the toxins don't get "stuck" in the body.

Silver Sol

Many use colloidal silver for killing infections. While it can be helpful for viral, bacterial, fungal, etc. infections, colloidal silver can also kill the good bacteria in the gut, and has the risk of Argyria (the permanent bluish tint of the skin from taking prolonged, high doses of colloidal silver). Silver sol is the safe alternative. It is an engineered nanoparticle rather than a colloid. Silver sol works as a catalyst to kill bacteria. It has the same wavelength frequency as germicidal ultraviolet light. Silver sol also spares the good bacteria in the gut so it can be taken safely on a long term basis. It also does not have the risk of Argyria, as the silver content is much lower than a colloidal silver. The lesser dose of silver does not mean that it is less effective than colloidal silver, in fact it has been proven to be more effective! After researching the differences between colloidal silver and silver sol, I only recommend using silver sol, and I would never use colloidal silver.

Nutrition

I also use a procedure to test the Kreb Cycle (how the body takes nutrients and converts them into energy for bodily functions). This helps to determine the nutritional need of the body while one is going through serial remedies. I use targeted nutritional and mineral support to give the body the specific nutrients it needs so that it has the energy to "fight" the infection. It is really a two part approach that I take. I use the serial remedies to give the body the information it needs and then use the Kreb Cycle testing to make sure the body has the nutrition and energy it needs to fight!

It's amazing how much better clients feel during serial remedies if they have the proper nutrients and nutrition and follow the recommendations I make! In order for a supplement to make it onto my shelf, it has been under intense scrutiny and has to contain quality natural ingredients and not synthetic vitamins.

I have had clients try to substitute with low quality supplements from big-box retailers only to complain how poorly they feel at their next appointment. At my practice, I don't use a one-size-fits-all protocol. I test each individual person to find what "their body" needs. I would emphasize, no two cases are identical, which is why modern medicine struggles so much with Lyme in particular. This individualized care takes time, but it is the most effective way to support the body during this process.

Chapter 6: Diet and Lifestyle Modifications

Bacteria feed on sugar and also foods that turn into sugar in the body, such as carbohydrates. Because of this, I believe that changing diet while fighting Lyme disease or another chronic infection is <u>crucial</u>. Why would you keep feeding something with sugar while at the same time trying to rid the body of it?

At first it can seem overwhelming to change diet, but starting with small changes and continually making new positive changes will make a world of difference. We need to remove things that may be difficult for your body process and provide it with the true nourishment it actually needs! Our goal throughout this entire process is to strengthen your own body to fight off the challenges it faces.

The products found in the middle aisles of the average American grocery store are not foods that will truly nourish the body. They are food-like shapes laden with toxic chemicals, neurotoxins, artificial chemical flavorings and colors, as well as GMO foods (oils, corn syrup, sugar, soy, etc). These foods are fortified with synthetic vitamins often derived from petroleum products or other chemical sources.

When so many are eating the Standard American Diet (SAD) ☹, how can we wonder why disease is rampant in the Western World? Our bodies need whole foods, fresh vegetables, small amounts of fruit, healthy sources of protein and good fats to truly thrive. When the body is in a diseased state, it needs to be truly nourished, not poisoned numerous times per day! There is a reason that the body has become weakened and diseased, and diet plays an important role in that.

Personally, I had already started to make some good changes to my diet, but when I discovered that I was fighting Lyme, I made some drastic changes.

I adopted a very low grain diet, high in vegetables, minimal raw dairy, moderate protein, fruits in moderation, and small amounts of natural sweeteners. But despite these changes, I found I was struggling with frequent bouts of hypoglycemia.

I eventually transitioned over to a ketogenic diet/lifestyle. Very high in healthy fats, moderate protein, as many vegetables as I could eat, and very low in carbohydrates. This has truly been life changing!

We have been taught since the 1960's the flawed research done by Framingham. This research stated that eating a diet high in saturated fat would increase blood cholesterol levels and was the cause of heart disease. In 1992, Dr William Castelli, the director of the Framingham study, publically declared that saturated fat would do no such thing. His data showed that the more saturated fat, cholesterol and calories that a person at, the lower serum cholesterol levels were.

Contrary to what we have been taught for the last 60 years about fat in our diet, saturated fats like coconut oil, butter, avocados, olives, etc. do not raise blood cholesterol or contribute to atherosclerosis. Sugars, sweeteners, and carbohydrates cause inflammation which raises cholesterol and can cause coronary artery disease. Cholesterol in proper amounts is a good and necessary thing. Cholesterol is a protective mechanism that the body uses when there is inflammation and it needs help with healing. If I cut my finger, my body will send cholesterol to the site of the cut to assist with the healing process. So why do so many have heart disease and atherosclerosis? Stop and think about the Standard American Diet ☹, where we've been taught to eat a high carbohydrate diet, as much sugar as we want, just don't eat too much fat. Could the inflammation in the blood vessels be due to the high sugar content in the blood spiking numerous times per day caused by this diet? Could the inflammation also be due to a chronic infection that has never been identified? I believe that these things are a key underlying cause of heart disease and atherosclerosis.

Along with this ketogenic diet I have done some fasting and the hypoglycemia that I had for years is gone. I now intermittent fast 6 days a week for about 18 hours per day. This means I eat dinner at about 6PM and then don't eat any solid food the next day until around noon. In the morning I use some oils (healthy fats) to help balance my blood sugar. I put a tablespoon of butter and a tablespoon of MCT oil in my coffee in the morning. I can then wait until noon before eating with no issues! Some days if I am busy, I don't eat until close to 2PM. The reason this works so well is because I have converted my body from burning sugar (when I would have to eat every 2-3 hours and still suffer hypoglycemia in between) to burning fat. Contrary to what we have all been taught for so many years, carbohydrates (sugars) are not essential for brain function. When the body burns fat or stored fat, it produces ketones which are another fuel for the brain to run on. The most amazing thing about this process is how ketones help to heal the brain. I suffered for a while with significant brain fog, but since transitioning to the ketogenic diet and eliminating the Lyme infection, I feel my brain is so much clearer. Chronic Lyme can cause many issues with the brain not functioning properly so I believe that it's important to use any tools you can to help heal the brain. Ketones burn much cleaner than glucose or sugar in body. The waste products produced by burning glucose are much more difficult for the body to process than those produced by burning fats.

Now, I do understand that there are significant differences in the way each person is able to handle foods. Each body is different and I don't think there is just one diet for everyone. Some may do better with a Paleo type diet rather than a Ketogenic diet. It's important to listen to your body while experimenting and working with an experienced practitioner.

I now crave whole, fresh, real food that has nutritional value. I no longer have any desire to eat at popular chain restaurants that we used to frequent. Even back then, I would wonder why my fingers were swollen, why I was incredibly thirsty and would feel "yucky" after eating there. I figured it out pretty quickly once I was completely off of the popular food additive Monosodium Glutamate (MSG). These symptoms were from the MSG that was added to much of the food. People have gone into these popular chain restaurants and asked to order something from the menu that didn't contain MSG, and have been told that there is nothing on the menu that doesn't contain MSG. Even the salad dressing has it! MSG is a potent neurotoxin that alters the brain and actually makes the body want to eat more. This is so important to avoid!

I search out restaurants that offer healthier options, and the taste is exceptional compared to the popular chain restaurants. I feel so much better after eating real food, rather than food like objects flavored with artificial flavors, preservatives, GMOs and MSG. I do realize that this makes it harder to live a so called "normal" life, but if you truly care about the one body you have, you must consider it.

Lifestyle Changes

It's important to evaluate your lifestyle. The typical stressful, busy American lifestyle doesn't allow time for the body to heal.

Try to evaluate stress load and reduce this as much as possible. Lyme changes your priorities and things that used to matter don't matter as much anymore when your lifestyle becomes one focused on survival. We live in such a materialistic society and when you are forced to step back and look at what truly matters, your priorities start to change.

Stress affects the immune system. Slow down and listen to the birds on a morning walk, appreciate the beautiful sunrises on the drive to work in the morning. Step outside and breathe. Look and listen to how quiet the world is when the snowflakes are falling. Learn to appreciate beauty in every season!

Sleep

Having a chronic infection often affects the ability to sleep or stay asleep. It is advisable to get at least 8 hours of sleep per night to allow the body to rest and heal. This can be extremely frustrating when not able to stay asleep due to the infections. Feeling exhausted during the day but wide awake, unable to sleep during the night. Yes, I've been there!

We made changes to our bedtime as an attempt to get enough sleep. It may not work for everyone, but we try to go to bed at around 8:30PM every night. It helps to be on a schedule and to stay on that schedule during the weekend also if possible. The hours between 10PM – 2AM are the most valuable hours of sleep for physical healing. The more sleep you can get between those hours, the better!

Personally I have found that toxicity has been a major factor that affected my sleep. Taking measures to address the toxicity in the body makes a huge difference. Parasites can also present a challenge. Taking the correct anti-parasitic herbs or homeopathic remedies can control and eliminate this problem. Without them, the little "critters" can interfere with the ability to get to sleep and stay asleep throughout the night.

Magnesium deficiency can cause sleep challenges as well. Supplementing with Magnesium right before bedtime can help with sleep and prevent cramping during the middle of the night.

Amazingly, magnetic therapy using a PEMF machine (see Chapter 7) dramatically helped improve my sleep while I was fighting the infections. Since the first few days of using the machine, my sleep has been deep and restful.

Chapter 7: Helpful Tools to Ease Clearing Reactions

Throughout my journey with Lyme and other chronic infections, I accumulated some helpful tools to ease detox or clearing reactions while going through the homeopathic process.

I am not a medical doctor, and therefore anything I say should not be taken as medical advice. Before starting anything yourself, you should consult with your healthcare provider or practitioner.

Epsom Salt Bath

I struggled with muscle pain in my shoulders and neck while using homeopathy to clear infections. I would at times have significant joint pain as well, but that cleared up much more quickly than the muscle pain.

I found that it was helpful to use Epsom Salt baths with some relaxing essential oils added. These were easy to do and the magnesium helped relax and ease the muscle pain. The detoxification even helped me with some of the brain fog. Soaking in warm water helps draw toxins out through the skin and therefore take some of the burden of detoxification off of the kidneys and liver.

For a while I would do a bath 2-3 times per week, but

some people even do them every day.

To prepare the bath,

-Fill tub with enough warm water that will cover most of your body.

-Dissolve 1 ½ cups of Epsom salts for an adult weighing over 100lbs, 1 cup of Epsom salts for a child weighing 60-100lbs, and ½ cup Epsom salts for a child weighing under 60lbs.

-Add 1/2 cup of baking soda if on city water with chlorine.

-Essential oils of your choice (optional), I usually add some lavender for relaxation.

Soak in the tub for about 20 minutes and then rinse off after the bath. Make time to rest after the bath, because it can make you feel pretty exhausted. I prefer to do the bath an hour before bedtime.

Infrared Heating Pad

One of the most effective products I have tried and one that helped me through the healing process and reduced my discomfort was an infrared heating pad. It is important to purchase from a reputable company and not just any knock off. I have a brand that I prefer and recommend to my clients.

Warning, I would never use a regular heating pad on myself or recommend that anyone else use one. Heating pads use coils inside that emit high amounts of EMF (Electromagnetic Fields/Electromagnetic Radiation). This radiation emitted is invisible to the eye, but putting something like this directly against parts of your body causes high amounts of stress to the body and has been shown to increase risk of cancer. We are exposed to too much EMF in our daily life already from WI-FI, cell phones, bluetooth, etc., without placing a heating pad directly over our body. If you have one of the regular heating pads, I recommend getting rid of it or not using it, the same goes for electric blankets. A good quality infrared healing pad emits very low to almost no EMF. It is the safe alternative to a regular heating pad.

Infrared Heating Pads offer the following benefits:

-Penatrating heat that warms and relaxes muscles and tissues
-Increases blood circulation to the area
-Reduction in stress and fatigue

The owner of the company I buy my infrared heating pads from designed the products and started his company to help his daughter as she was going through Lyme disease treatment. In no way do I believe that this is the only thing you can use to "kill the Lyme", though the hyperthermia could have some effect on the infection. I used it more to ease some of the reactions that occur during the healing process.

On the days that I would wake up feeling the intense muscle pain, I would use the infrared heating pad for

20-60 minutes. It relieved the pain enough that I would be able to function reasonably well the rest of the day. It would literally "melt away my muscle pain". Some days I would use the heating pad twice per day, after being at work or on my feet all day.

Sauna

My husband and I built our own near infrared sauna. The sauna works in numerous ways to help you through the detoxification process. First, it heats the body, which is helpful since most people with a Lyme infection have low body temperature. The infrared heat penetrates several inches deep, into the body and causes the body to go through the same physiological process as it would if running 5 miles. Because the body heats up, it causes vasodilation as the body tries to cool itself, this induces sweating, increases heart rate, etc.

A near infrared sauna is different than a steam sauna that you may find at health clubs or fitness centers. A steam sauna uses very hot air to heat the body from the outside in, but without the infrared the heat isn't able to penetrate the body. Many individuals complain of feeling uncomfortable or unable to breathe in a steam sauna due to the high temperature. A near infrared sauna uses infrared heat bulbs that heat the air, but also penetrate the body several inches deep.

Second, because of the sweating, the pores open up and the skin creates another route of detoxification. Many people with Lyme disease or chronic infections have a lowered body temperature and don't sweat much. This helps to raise the core body temperature. One of the strangest things that happened in our personal experience were the smells that came from the sweat wiped off with a rag during sauna use. While going through the homeopathic serial remedies for Lyme, we noticed that there was a very strong ammonia smell that would come from our sweat. This is interesting because ammonia is a byproduct released from the destruction of the Borrelia bacteria. When getting to the end of dealing with the Lyme, we noticed the ammonia smell had lessened considerably.

When doing saunas, it is extremely important to be well hydrated prior to the sauna, and then drink plenty of fluids after. It is also helpful to supplement with a minerals. I find that my body craves salt after a sauna, so I place about 1 tsp of Himalyan salt in a glass of water and drink that.

It is also very important to start slowly with saunas. If you are not used to sweating very often or your body doesn't sweat at all when it is warm, it is important to go slow and gradually work up the time in the sauna. I personally started with about 15 minutes, and slowly worked my way up to 30 minutes. Some people find that they are able to do a

40-60 minute sauna, but I find that even 30 minutes is long enough. If I tried to stay in much longer than that, I would feel worse, and extremely fatigued. Be in tune with your body and listen to it on how it is reacting to different things. If you aren't interested in building your own sauna, the company I purchase my infrared heating pads from makes one that I would recommend. It has Near, Mid and Far Infrared heat, EMF protected and is quite portable. Be cautious when purchasing a sauna as to what materials (chemical sealers or glues) might be used in it's construction. You don't want to increase your exposure to more toxins.

Saunas should not be used by pregnant women, children under the age of 10 and should always be supervised with older children, people with heart problems, and high blood pressure. Always check with your healthcare provider prior to starting sauna therapy.

Chiropractic

I found chiropractic care during the process of fighting infection to be very beneficial for me. The days after an adjustment I found I would sleep better and have more energy. Chiropractic care focuses on the health of the nervous system and removing blockages (subluxation). Remember what I mentioned before, our bodies are designed to heal, they just need the interference removed.

Massage

I also found that massage was helpful for me to relax my muscles. I tended to have pain and muscle soreness in my upper back and neck while going through the protocols to heal from the infections. Massage was wonderful to relax those muscles and give me some relief from the pain. Use caution with massage if your body is not detoxing well, it may release too many toxins. Start with a gentle massage, not deep tissue and see how your body handles that. Make sure to stay well-hydrated before and after!

Craniosacral Therapy

Contrary to what is taught in American medical colleges, our cranial bones do not fuse together in adulthood.

Craniosacral Therapy has been taught by John Upledger and by palpating the cranial bones, one can feel the rhythmic pulsing of the cranial bones due to the pressure of the cerebral spinal fluid and arterial pressure. By palpating, one can feel if there are disturbances in the pulses and very light pressure can be used to bring the pulsing back into balance. From personal experience of having Craniosacral therapy done, at first I wondered if it was actually going to do anything. The pressure by the therapist is very light and subtle. It was extremely relaxing and the following day, I would feel like I had a spinal adjustment, I slept better, and had more energy.

PEMF (Pulsed Electromagnetic Field Therapy)

An exciting therapy that we have also been using is called Pulsed Electromagnetic Field Therapy (PEMF). PEMF therapy devices use a control unit to administer pulsed magnetic fields to the body using various applicators such as a full body mat and localized applicators.

PEMF therapy helps to recharge the cells in our bodies. It helps to increase circulation and oxygenation, increases ATP production, helps the cells get rid of toxins and be able to get nutrients into the cells.

A good way of looking at healthy cells in our bodies is to think of a grape. These grapelike cells swell and contract slightly, allowing nutrients in and toxins out. When the cells become unhealthy due to toxin exposure, infections, and poor diet, these cells start to look more like shriveled raisins. The membrane around the cell becomes inflamed and no longer lets a proper amount of nutrients in or toxins out. This can cause extreme fatigue, the immune system can no longer fight infections properly, the body continues to become more and more toxic, and this is a basis for developing cancer, etc.

There are 4 main things that help to regenerate the cell membrane and cell health and help the cell go from raisin-like to grape-like again! Raw, healthy food, spring water, exercise and PEMF. The first three are very slow in rejuvenating the cells. I have seen this personally in my husband. Despite eating a near perfect diet for years, taking the highest quality supplements, he continued to be fatigued, had low cellular energy, was not able to fight off infections, etc. He was unable to exercise, although active at his job, because of the fatigue, it took everything he had just to continue working.

Pain and discomfort are signs of cellular imbalance and disease. Cellular Exercise is a safe and effective way to support cellular energy needs and has been shown to help with the following:

- Support Healthy Cellular Function
- Stimulates exchange of cellular fluids
- Speed up the body's self-healing ability
- Reduce pain and inflammation
- Relieve injury and fatigue
- Reduce stress and increase relaxation
- Achieve a deeper, more restorative sleep

Each cell in our body has a power center called the mitochondria. The function of the mitochondria is to produce energy or voltage (ATP). Therefore, each cell in our body has electrical energy. This is acknowledged by conventional medicine when taking an EKG of the heart. The EKG measures the electrical activity of the heart. Or an EEG of the brain, measuring the electrical activity of the brain.

When there is disease, the voltage in the cells falls to less than half of the required voltage. Thus, the body can't produce healthy new cells and disease and symptoms manifest. PEMF exercises the cells and helps them to again produce this necessary energy.

I cannot make any claims that PEMF therapy will cure or treat disease, but it is used to energize the body, so that the body can do what it is designed to do, heal. It has been incredibly helpful to me and my practice. While perhaps it is not a necessity for all of my clients, it has proven to be very beneficial for those struggling the most. It can also be beneficial for those struggling with back and knee pain, inflammation, assists with post-surgical healing and broken bones as it helps stimulate tissues to regenerate and heal more quickly. Some have avoided surgery by using PEMF therapy.

Chapter 8: Discovering Impairments in the Immune System and the Reason Chronic Infections Took Hold - Heavy Metals, Toxins, etc.

Immune system impairments can range from stress, to toxic foods, chemicals, heavy metals, infections, etc.

It is important to look at your lifestyle and evaluate why your immune system was not able to fight off a chronic infection. What other dysfunction is going on?

Toxins

We live in an extremely toxic world. More toxic than ever before. The chemicals we are exposed to on a daily basis are affecting the way our bodies function. There are 70,000 chemicals produced in North America alone. 1,000 new chemicals are produced each year. Testing is minimal and yet we use them with little to no study of the consequences.

There are 70,000 food additives that have been approved by the FDA. These range from genetically modified foods, to artificial flavors, to preservatives. They inundate our food supply! Most of these additives have never truly been studied, or the studies for safety have been performed by the manufacturer, which quite possibly did not result in an unbiased study.

GMO's, or genetically modified organisms, are plants, animals, microorganisms or other organisms whose genetic makeup has been modified using recombinant DNA methods (also called gene splicing), gene modification or transgenic technology. They have not been proven to be safe for consumption by people or animals. In addition to the genetic modifications of the seeds and plants, GMO corn, soy, sugar beets, etc. are all sprayed with glyphosate (the ingredient in herbicide). Studies have shown that glyphosate separates the tight junctions in the gut, basically tearing microscopic holes in the gut. This can cause something called leaky gut. A good way to envision this is to think of a fishing net. In a healthy gut (fishing net) only certain things are able to pass through the membrane into the blood stream. When the gut/fishing net gets holes in it; larger particles like undigested food, chemicals, toxins, can pass directly into the blood stream. These large particles cause the immune system to react because they aren't supposed to be there. This in turn causes constant low grade inflammation throughout the body. When the immune system is over-stimulated in this way, it starts to over-react to everyday particles, causing allergies or intolerance symptoms. This can also lead to auto-immunity when the body is no longer able distinguish it's own cells and those of foreign invaders. This chronic inflammation takes over and increases the risk of developing all chronic diseases.

Another concern is BT toxin (Bacillus Thuringiensis) in some GMO crops; sugar beets, corn, squash, and cotton. BT is an insecticide and these plants have been genetically engineered to produce this toxin. When the insect starts to feed on the crop, the ingested BT breaks open the stomach and kills it. So, if BT does this to insects, what happens when people start to eat food with these GMO ingredients?

A study was carried out by independent doctors at the University of Sherbrooke Hospital Centre in Quebec, Canada. They studied 30 pregnant women and 39 other women who were not pregnant. In the blood of 28 out of the 30 pregnant women, traces of BT toxin were found, equaling 93%. And traces of BT toxin were also found in the umbilical cords of 24 out of the 30 babies, 80%. In the group of women who weren't pregnant, traces of BT toxin were found in 27 out of 39 women. The researchers who performed this study stated that more research needed to be done as it appears that the BT toxin was able to cross the placenta and into a baby. There needs to be more studies done on the host of potential problems that BT toxin could cause.

We need to stop accepting GMOs in our food supply as safe, when the studies have not been done and the few independent studies that have been performed show that rats and mice that are fed a GMO diet develop tumors and cancer, kidney problems, liver problems, immune system problems, etc.

Stress

Stress can be overwhelming. Many times we don't think we have control over stressors; jobs, illness, and outside influences in our lives. It is important to find healthy ways of managing our stress. Mental and emotional stress is a great challenge to our immune system; it places pressure on nearly every organ system in the body. We need to be in tune with our body, listen to the warning signs and take measures to correct them before they manifest as symptoms of stress. Practice some relaxation techniques, deep breathing, gentle exercise like taking a walk. Giving time for plenty of sleep, positive thoughts and prayer. While working on healing the body, sometimes it is necessary to say no to nonessential things and focus on taking the time to heal! You only get one body, how you use it is entirely up to you.

Heavy Metals

Heavy metals cause a different kind of stress on the body, chemical stress. Heavy metals include lead, mercury, aluminum, arsenic, etc. Any metal that accumulates in the body and is difficult to remove once deposited in tissues, the brain, nervous system, or organs. Heavy metals enter our body through various avenues; congenital transmission, breathing, eating, vaccination, and absorption through the skin. Heavy metals are everywhere in our world. Lead was used in paint until the 1970's and used in gasoline in some places until the 1980's. Lead is still found in glazes on <u>new</u> kitchen dishes, drinking glasses, china, leaded crystal, toys, and many other things. Once you start to learn these things, your thinking changes and you begin to look at everything! But, it's a good change. I look at things in a completely different way now that I understand these things. I can make better, more informed choices to protect myself from ingesting lead and other toxins. You would think in our modern, more informed world it would be less of a challenge to make these safer, better choices. Don't make the mistake of assuming that if a product is offered for sale, it must be safe, good, and healthy for you. Only you can make this determination with certainty. This thought pattern applies whether it be food, supplements, medicine, or products you may use on a daily basis.

I believe I was exposed to lead from before birth,

throughout childhood and into adulthood. I have taken steps to remove the lead from my body by using chelation. Chelation comes from the Greek word – "chele" meaning claw. Chelation is using a chelating agent that binds with a metal or toxin so that it loses its toxic effect. It is a slow, sometimes uncomfortable process. Removing metals can cause symptoms of fatigue, headaches, and flaring of Candida infection symptoms. In the last number of years I have come to realize that some more natural practitioners believe that every symptom is caused by heavy metal toxicity and that's what they address first with their clients. Believing any other challenges/infections will clear up after the toxicity is dealt with. Through personal experience and working with clients I firmly believe that when the infection is the priority, the body does not have the energy or resources to do chelation as well. Heavy metal chelation should only be done when the body is ready. Also, when the body is given the nutrients and minerals it needs, it will naturally detoxify many heavy metals and doesn't always need to be forced with harsh chelators.

Lead has a molecularly similar structure to calcium, so when lead is ingested and the bones need calcium, it is stored within the bones. It is estimated that it takes about 2-4 years for the bone cells in your body to regenerate and completely rebuild your bones, so chelation can take some time. There are periods of time that more calcium is needed by the body and is taken from the bones, and usually the lead is released first. Puberty, pregnancy, and menopause are all life changes that tend to be times that lead is released from the bones at a faster rate. Lead most often deposits into the brain, bones, liver, kidneys and spleen. It is able to alter our behavior and intelligence and has been shown to significantly decrease intellectual development. Even when blood levels of lead are below current federal guidelines of 10mcg/dL this can produce a surprising drop in IQ of 7.4 points!

Mercury is a potent neurotoxin and is one of the most deadly substances known to man. It deposits in the brain, nervous system, kidneys, adrenals, heart, and other endocrine glands.

Oddly enough, mercury is found most commonly in amalgam fillings, they contain 51% mercury. Amalgam fillings are placed directly into the tooth tissue and can release mercury into the nerve root of the tooth. When someone has an amalgam filling, every time that person chews, drinks hot or cold liquids, or grinds teeth at night, mercury gas is released from the amalgam filling. Being in close proximity to the brain, this can have some pretty severe effects. Many degenerative neurological problems can be tied to mercury poisoning; these include memory loss, senility, tremors, and heart attacks. Mercury particularly affects the neurological system, the brain and the nerves. It also has been found that people with more amalgam fillings have more kidney function problems. Mercury likes to lodge in the kidneys and causes damage to kidney function.

Mercury has also been a preservative in contact lens wetting solution until the 1990's, used as a preservative in IV solutions and other pharmaceuticals, and is used as a preservative in vaccines.

Aluminum causes significant oxidative damage to the central nervous system; it also targets the cerebellum and the autonomic nervous system (which controls the activity in our bodies that happens 'automatically' meaning, we don't think about. For example, we don't think about breathing every 5-8 seconds, it is controlled by our autonomic nervous system. We don't think about digesting the food we just ate, or that our heart needs to pump 60-80 beats per minute.)

Aluminum is the most common vaccine adjuvant. The aluminum is added to vaccines to enhance the immune response to the antigen that is injected with the vaccine. Unfortunately, aluminum also impairs the body's ability to detoxify by reducing glutathione activity. Glutathione is called the master antioxidant. It is an important part of the detoxification process because it changes a harmful substance in the body into a less harmful one that can then be eliminated through the liver and bowel. So what does this all mean? By injecting a vaccine containing aluminum into the body, the aluminum enhances the immune response to the vaccine. This sounds like it should be a good thing, but the aluminum is also causing oxidative damage to the central nervous system. The aluminum impairs the body's ability to detoxify because the glutathione activity is impaired. The aluminum accumulates in the body and continues to cause degeneration of the nervous system.

Aluminum is also found in many foods, baking powder, salt, infant formula, drugs, cosmetics, and processed foods.

It's been found that cooking in or with aluminum foil or eating foods that are from aluminum containers, greatly increases our exposure. Think about what happens when acidic foods are in contact with aluminum foil. The acids can cause the foil to disintegrate into the food where it is likely to be ingested later.

I changed how I cook my food and will not use aluminum foil anymore. I simply use a clear glass baking dish with a glass lid. It's very practical and I use the glass cover instead of foil to cover the food I am cooking or later string in the refrigerator. Knowledge can bring about easy, positive changes!

There are other metals that can cause many different issues and it's important to find an experienced practitioner that can help guide you through testing and a heavy metal chelation program when needed. These metals are dangerous and if a chelation program is not done properly, can cause worsening of symptoms and possibly damage to the organs of the body. Simply taking some chlorella or cilantro is not proper chelation of heavy metals. Chlorella and cilantro have their place during chelation with other products, but they are very weak binders to toxins and metals. They will stir things up, but not bind to the metal and remove it from the body. It will most likely deposit in a different area or organ of the body. This is called retoxing, not detoxing!

If you have amalgam fillings in your mouth, don't just run out to your regular dentist and have them all removed. It is extremely important to find a biological dentist that does safe amalgam removal. This includes using a rubber dam to prevent pieces of the amalgam filling from going into the patient, using a fresh source of oxygen for the patient, covering the patient with a disposable cloth that is removed after the amalgam is out, using a special air filter to suck all of the mercury vapor out of the room, etc. Work with a practitioner prior to having amalgam fillings removed to be on a good detoxification program and get the body ready in the few months leading up to and after the removal. There are steps and processes that should be followed to minimized the exposure before, during and after the removal.

Why did I go so in depth with Heavy metals in a Lyme and chronic infection book? Lyme infection and heavy metals are commonly seen together. As I stated before, metals weaken and impair the immune system, cause damage to the liver, kidneys, heart, nervous system, endocrine glands and brain. This weakened condition allow infections to take hold more readily.

Pyroluria

Pyroluria is believed to be a genetic condition that causes the liver to overproduce pyrroles when hemoglobin is broken down. Pyroluria is also known as Kryptopyrroluria (KPU) or Hemopyrrollactamuria (HPU) and more specifically as hydroxyhemoppyrrolin-2-one or HPL. A long time ago was known as the "mauve factor". Pyroluria has been known in the psychiatric world since the 1950's when Abram Hoffer MD, PhD was looking for a biochemical origin in schizophrenia. The "mauve factor" would be found in the urine of schizophrenic patients and not in the control group. Throughout the years various doctors have found that when these schizophrenic patients were given high doses of vitamin B6 and zinc their condition improved. Even though this has been recognized by psychiatrists for many decades, most doctor medical associations do not recognize it because there are no pharmaceuticals that treat it, only supplements. Most likely your medical doctor has never heard of it.

Why do I mention this? Dr. Klinghardt found a correlation between his patients with Lyme disease and pyroluria. He found the incidence of pyroluria in Lyme disease patients to be 80% or higher. He also found it in patients with heavy metal toxicity. More than 75% of children with Autism tested positive for pyroluria as well.

There is research that indicates that pyroluria is a genetic condition that can run in families. About 10-15% of people suffer from this, and symptoms worsen over a person's lifetime, even more with stress. There is also an environmental factor as the onset frequently occurs during a stressful event in late teens or early adulthood. It can be triggered by injury, mental stress, infections, illness, or toxin exposure.

I mention this because in April 2016, I listened to a Lyme disease webinar and the speaker started talking about pyroluria. She started describing the symptoms of it and I listened very intently. She was describing me! I could identify with SOOOO many of the symptoms, things that I hadn't been able to understand or discover the cause of. The most notable was extreme anxiety when I would go to an appointment or do anything out of the ordinary. The anxiety was so extreme that I would be inwardly trembling. My hands and body would be sweating and I couldn't focus or think. These appointments would be simply going to an eye doctor, or seeing a naturopath. Not scary events, it wasn't like I was having surgery or anything. I kept thinking to myself "I'm a nurse, why am I feeling this way?" It wasn't an anxiety related to fearfulness. It was something that was physiologically wrong with my body!

Common symptoms or conditions related to Pyroluria are Lyme disease, allergies to foods or environment, acne, cold hands and feet, crowded teeth (prior to orthodontic treatment), reduced hair on head and eyebrows, nervous exhaustion, severe inner tension, low stress tolerance, tendency to avoid large groups of people or new situations, travel is particularly stressful, fatigue, dry skin, insomnia, inability to recall dreams, poor memory in general, poor tolerance of alcohol or medications – a little produces a strong response, increased sensitivity to sound, light, smells and touch, digestive issues, poor appetite, especially in the morning, more alert and capable in the evening, got a stitch in the side when running as a child, irregular menstrual periods, joint pain in the knees or legs, creaking joints, motion sickness, weakened immune system causing chronic bacterial, fungal or viral infections.
A simple urine test will detect if this is a problem.

Vitamin B6, Zinc, Biotin and Omega 6 are supplements that are important remedies for Pyroluria. For Vitamin B6 - look for the active form called pyridoxal 5'-phosphate (P5P) versus the inactive form pyridoxine. Some may do better with a combination of P5P and pyridoxine.

It is important to work with a practioner on supplementation. Taking high doses of Vitamin B6 can pull magnesium from the body creating a deficiency, therefore magnesium supplementation needs to be addressed. When higher dose zinc supplementation is started, it can cause the body to "dump" heavy metals very quickly. This needs to be managed with a heavy metal chelation program along with antioxidant supplementation. As you can see, it is more complicated than just taking high dose Vitamin B6 and Zinc supplements. Everything in the body works together and needs to be balanced!

Also, because the pyroles bind to omega-6 fatty acids, it's important to get enough good sources of omega-6 using diet. Eggs, red meat, liver, butter, black currant seed oil and evening primrose oil are all good sources.

Chapter 9: Supporting Various Organs and Systems in the Body During and After the Homeopathic Protocols

While working to heal from a chronic infection like Lyme or other co-infection, it is important to look for imbalances in the other organ systems of the body. Lyme and other infections cause many imbalances in the body that lead to dysfunction.

Fighting a long term infection can cause adrenal fatigue, thyroid imbalances, liver congestion, leaky gut, etc.

Adrenal Fatigue

The adrenal glands are what manage stress in the body. They are responsible for producing cortisol when there is stress on the body. This stress could be from chronic infection, inflammation, pain, emotional stress or physical stress such as exposure to extreme temperatures. It is a normal thing for the adrenals to produce cortisol when the body is exposed to these stressors. The problem occurs when the stress becomes chronic and doesn't go away. The adrenal glands then have to work harder and harder to continue to produce cortisol. Over time, this mechanism breaks down and the adrenal glands are unable to produce the necessary amount of cortisol.

This can lead to feelings of total mental, physical and emotional exhaustion. When cortisol levels are low in the body, the body will become more inflamed and the person can experience more pain.

While dealing with a Lyme infection, adrenal support is often necessary. There are various alternative ways of testing for adrenal fatigue and working with an experienced practitioner is always recommended.

There are many different nourishing herbs, tinctures and homeopathic remedies that I have personally used and now recommend for adrenal support during and after Lyme protocols. B Vitamin Complex, especially one with pantothenic acid (vitamin B5), and Vitamin C can also help with adrenal function. Eating a healthy diet that is low in inflammatory foods can also be very beneficial. Avoid gluten, corn, sugar, and dairy. These foods are all very inflammatory. Also try to eat a lower carbohydrate diet. Eating a large amount of carbohydrates makes blood sugar spike, thus increasing insulin production and a blood sugar drop. This process drives inflammation. It is very stressful on the adrenal glands to have these large blood sugar spikes and crashes. Switching to a ketogenic diet is very beneficial for some. (See Chapter 5 for more information on ketogenic diet)

Liver Congestion

The liver is the detox or filtration organ for our blood. When there is a chronic infection in the body, the blood becomes sticky. It doesn't flow as well as it should throughout the body. With a chronic infection like Lyme, the liver is likely to be congested. The liver can process only so many toxins and what it cannot process, the body stores away for processing later. These toxins are mainly stored in the fat of the body. When there is a co-infection like Bartonella, the liver and spleen are usually enlarged. Sometimes the gallbladder is involved as well. Using homeopathic and herbal supplements that help the liver with drainage and other actions can be very helpful.
Milk thistle is especially protective of the liver from microbial or chemical toxins. It can help with the regeneration of a damaged liver and also tone and normalize liver function. When milk thistle is used in combination with red root, it helps to stimulate bile flow and production.

Mitochondrial Dysfunction

Each cell in our body has a "powerhouse" called the mitochondria. These "powerhouses" help to produce our energy. This production of energy is also called ATP (adenosine triphosphate). When the body has been sick for an extended period of time, exposed to chemicals, toxic metals, toxic foods and oils, etc. the cell membrane (the layer surrounding the outside of the cell), becomes unable to let the good nutrients into the cell and unable to let the bad toxins out of the cell. Thus, the "powerhouse", mitochondria inside the cell isn't able to produce the energy that it should because it can't get the nutrients it needs. This is a large factor in the fatigue that is felt when very ill with chronic infections.

To begin repairing the Mitochondria and the membrane, the first step is to remove the source of the toxins.

Then, the focus needs to be on repairing the membrane of the cell. Cut out french fries, chips, and vegetable oils from the diet. These toxic oils take about 60 days for the body to process and eliminate! Instead the body needs healthy fats from butter, coconut oil, cold pressed sesame oil, grass fed meats, avocados, olives, etc. Some other nutrients that nourish and heal the cell membrane are fat soluble antioxidants, tocotrienols, CoQ10, and lipoic acid.

See PEMF info in Chapter 6 for more info.

Thyroid Dysfunction

When a person has adrenal dysfunction, there can also quite commonly be thyroid dysfunction. Remember, all the systems in the body work together, when one breaks down, it causes a cascading effect on other systems that have to now work harder to maintain balance or homeostasis in the body. The adrenals, thyroid, pituitary, and hypothalamus all work together.

Lyme or other chronic infections, namely Epstein Barr, can have profound effects on the thyroid gland. The thyroid is quite susceptible to autoimmune issues and Lyme can be a trigger for autoimmune responses in the body.

It is important to work with an experienced practitioner if a thyroid imbalance is suspected. There are many things that need to be considered before just taking any supplement that you can purchase yourself. There are some very helpful homeopathics and supplementing with iodine can be beneficial as well. If you are supporting the thyroid, you also need to look at adrenal function support. Every system is connected.

Musculoskeletal System Pain

Most people with Lyme disease and other co-infections have some form of joint or muscle pain. No two people experience symptoms of Lyme the same way so the pain can be varied. While undergoing protocols to deal with the infection, it is important to manage the pain as best you can. I personally don't recommend taking narcotic pain medication and try to stay away from pharmaceuticals. This is an individual decision, but I have found some wonderful natural products that have worked for me.

Magnesium is a relaxant to the skeletal muscles and can provide some relief from painful, tight, cramping, aching muscles. Epsom salt baths can be very useful and relaxing. Epsom salts contain magnesium sulfate. Magnesium is also an effective therapy for constipation, although I believe you should find the true cause of the constipation (in some people it could be Magnesium deficiency!).

I have tried various different herbal anti-inflammatory supplements and have found some that work very well. A few that help with joint and muscle pain are white willow bark, boswellia, curcumin, and ginger.

I have also found some help from proteolytic enzymes which help to break down some of the chemical mediator and tissue by-products of inflammation. These are not meant to be taken as digestive enzymes, they should be taken on an empty stomach so that they help with the inflammation, rather than be used to digest food. Take the enzymes at least ½ hour prior to eating or at least 2 hours after eating. Some examples of proteolytic enzymes are bromelain, protease, and papain. I use a wonderful combination of these enzymes in a liposomal delivery system. Liposomal delivery means that small amounts of nutrients are bound to a fat cell taken from a high quality oil Phosphatidylcholine. It's an excellent way to deliver nutrients to the body because it bypasses the gut absorption of nutrients and due to the nature of the oil, the nutrients can pass directly into the blood stream. It is similar to getting an IV dose. The complaint with using proteolytic enzymes has always been that it takes a large amount of capsules to get a little bit of a result as many of the enzymes are broken down in the gut prior to being absorbed and used by the body to modulate the inflammation. Using a liposomal delivery form takes away the need to take large amounts of capsules.

I have also had some good results with various homeopathic pain remedies. These seem to work especially well when combined with some herbal products.

Nervous System

The pain that often accompanies a Lyme infection is different in every person. It can be a burning, shooting or stabbing pain. It can be either very debilitating or fairly mild.
Some of the other nervous system symptoms of Lyme disease include twitching of facial muscles and numbness in arms or legs.

Chapter 10: How to Live a Healthy Lifestyle, Investing in Your Future to Avoid Chronic Health Problems

How long will this process take to complete? It is truly impossible to say. Some respond quickly and others take longer, but I have seen amazing healing in both myself and my clients. The reason you are reading this is because there is no magic pill that you can take that will instantly make you better. It's a journey that has many ups and downs, one that takes time and commitment. Many practitioners say that it will take about 3 months of healing for every year that you've been sick. The body takes time to rebuild and heal. I am functioning so much better than I was a few years ago, truly thriving and feeling better than I ever remember feeling.

After the Lyme infection and other co-infections have been cleared and the immune system is functioning properly, it is very important to evaluate your lifestyle going forward. You probably had to make significant changes while dealing with the infections. What do you do now? Now is a great time to decide to implement permanent lifestyle changes to keep your immune system strong and healthy. I call it investing in your future. You only get one body and how are you going to care for it? I personally would like to live the healthiest life I possibly can. I never want to go back to the low point in my life when I could barely get out bed and was unable to do many normal activities.

What is the prognosis is for living a healthy life after Lyme and other chronic infections? We're in the first decades of dealing with these chronic infections, so there isn't a lot of information out there yet to answer that long term question.

The following are examples of how our body repairs damage and replaces old cells with new. Skin cells turn over about every 27 days, blood cells turn over every 3-4 months, muscle cells every 1-3 years, bone cells every 2-4 years, and nervous system every 7 years.

To me, these are very positive facts. I believe the body is designed to heal itself as long as it has the correct nutrients and the interference has been removed.

Lyme changed me in many ways, priorities have definitely changed. Many times during the difficult years, I would find myself feeling sorry for myself and longing for my old life back. Then I realized that I've changed, I wouldn't fit into my old life anymore. Things that used to be so important no longer are.

I've matured, I've changed and it is time to embrace these changes, live in the present and create a new life. Simplicity in life has become more important. I'm sure you've experienced changes as well.

Finding Balance In Life

It is important to find balance in life. One can get so over-committed and concerned with many things that truly are not important. There are pressures to do everything, and be everything to everyone. I grew up always being taught to put others first. That is an important way to live, but I've also learned that if I always put others first, I can become overwhelmed with everything, can't do anything to the best of my ability and become burned out. I learned the important lesson that I need to take care of myself as well so that I can help others. I understand the challenges of this, especially with Lyme and other chronic infections. On the outside, you may not look sick at all. There are no outward signs, no surgical scars, no broken bones that others understand. You may even have had Medical Doctors tell you that according to your blood work, you are the healthiest person they've seen! You may look completely normal, maybe a bit tired and worn at times. People may not realize the pain, fatigue and sorrow that goes on in your private life. Trust me, my husband and I know how you feel. We didn't tell many people of our struggles because of these reasons and simply because it was tiresome just trying to explain. During this whole ordeal, I'm sure we disappointed people by saying no to doing many different things. When you are fighting just to survive, you don't have the time or energy to do "normal" things, extra things. During that time I had to move past the expectations of others and focus on taking care of myself and my husband first.

It is a difficult thing to deal with emotionally when chronic illness drags on so long. But God had a plan for our lives and His plan is better than any plan we could ever come up with. The same is true for you! Seeing a doctor that had a history of Lyme himself also gave us hope. It was encouraging to see that he came through this experience himself and charted a course that we could follow. He is able to run a busy practice and is helping so many. We continue to be encouraged in seeing ourselves, friends and clients with similar conditions becoming well again. I believe we have been brought through this so we can provide this same hope for others.

Lastly, don't dwell on the negative. I understand if you are reading this, you or someone close to you has plenty to feel negative about. Resist it. I get tired of negativity around me, people complaining about the weather, or how this little thing or that little thing are not how they like it. Don't surround yourself with people like that. Find the good things that have been provided for you even during an incredibly difficult time. It can be very helpful to have a good friend to talk to, one that listens and doesn't judge.

Even when you have a really serious challenge like Lyme, stay positive because again, there is hope.

Conclusion

It is my hope and prayer that you can use the material contained in this book either for yourself or can pass it on to someone that can benefit from it. That what has been learned through a difficult experience is not wasted. My hope is to rescue those who are jumping from practitioner to practitioner, doctor to doctor, never finding adequate methods of testing or treatment, spending so much money with little to no results. I want to give someone hope that there are methods of dealing with chronic infections that don't involve years of antibiotics with still no result.

I hope to offer an "Alternative Approach". Showing that there is a way to bring the body back into balance, so the body can do what it has been created to do....heal.

My passion is to inspire you to take charge of your own health. No one is going to do this for you. You have to be the one to decide to change.

The change just might be worth it!

About Ashley

Ashley and her husband opened Alternative Approach Wellness Center in 2017. It is her passion to work with clients suffering from Lyme and chronic infections and to offer a different approach to healing the entire body. An individualized approach that values the innate intelligence of the body, determining the body's needs and not forcing the body to do what it isn't ready to do. Using this philosophy, she is seeing her clients healing and getting well faster than she hoped possible!

Thank you to our clients who have joined us on the road to better health!

www.alternativeapproachwellnesscenter.com

References

Chapter 1
Monogamous? This STD Doesn't Care, Melissa White

Healing Lyme, Stephen Harrod Buhner, 2015

The Beginner's Guide to Lyme Disease, Nicola McFadzean, N.D.

www.ilads.org

https://www.cdc.gov/lyme/stats/humancases.html

Chapter 2
Healing Lyme, Stephen Harrod Buhner, 2015

Magnarelli LA, Anderson JF, Barbour. The etiologic agent of Lyme disease in deer flies, horse flies, and mosquitos. AGJ Infect Dis. 1986 Aug;154(2):355-8

Magnarelli LA, Anderson JF. Ticks and biting insects infected with the etiologic agent of Lyme disease, Borrelia burgdorferi. J Clin Microbiol. 1988 Aug;26(8):1482-86

Monogamous? This STD Doesn't Care, Melissa White

The Beginner's Guide to Lyme Disease, Nicola

McFadzean, N.D.

https://www.cdc.gov/lyme/transmission/index.ht
ml

https://www.cdc.gov/mmwr/preview/mmwrhtml
/00038469.htm

Dressler F, et al. ANN INTERNAL MED. 1991.
115:533-539. Forsberg P, et al. CLIN EXP IMMUNOL.
1995; 101:453-460

http://holisticprimarycare.net/topics/topics-h-
n/infectious-disease/1512-new-t-cell-test-a-game-
changer-for-lyme-.html

Dr Myerowitz, D.C., Dilp. Ac. (NCCAOM), Lac.,
F.I.C.C., DABCA, BCIM speaker at DesBio 2016
Symposium, September 17th, 2016 (Reprinted with
permission)

Chapter 3
Healing Lyme, Stephen Harrod Buhner, 2015 pg 444

Dr Myerowitz, D.C., Dilp. Ac. (NCCAOM), Lac.,
F.I.C.C., DABCA, BCIM speaker at the DesBio 2016
Symposium

The Beginner's Guide to Lyme Disease, Nicola
McFadzean, N.D.

Mycoplasma Infections – DesBio articles November, 19th 2012

Chapter 4

https://www.researchgate.net/publication/2416974 25_Dynamics_of_connective-tissue_localization_during_chronic_Borrelia_burgdorferi_infection

https://bmcgenomics.biomedcentral.com/articles/1 0.1186/s12864-017-3553-5

Healing Lyme, Stephen Harrod Buhner, 2015

https://www.ncbi.nlm.nih.gov/pmc/articles/PMC2 515351/

http://bodyecology.com/articles/your-gut-can-influence-how-you-feel-it-all-starts-with-serotonin

https://www.priweb.org/ed/pgws/uses/vitamins.html

The Beginner's Guide to Lyme Disease, Nicola McFadzean, N.D.

Chapter 5

The Complete Guide to Homeopathy, The Principles and Practice of Treatment 1995, Dr. Andrew Lockie and Dr. Nicola Geddes

Dr Myerowitz, D.C., Dilp. Ac. (NCCAOM), Lac., F.I.C.C., DABCA, BCIM speaker at the DesBio 2016 Symposium 9/17/2016

Chapter 6
http://www.healthy-eatingpolitics.com/saturated-fats.html

http://www.niagara-gazette.com/news/lifestyles/natural-health-cholesterol-is-misunderstood/article_c0df483c-19ce-50f5-bd59-da4822b4b9bb.html

http://www.marksdailyapple.com/a-metabolic-paradigm-shift-fat-carbs-human-body-metabolism/

The Beginner's Guide to Lyme Disease, Nicola McFadzean, N.D.

Chapter 7
http://www.drlwilson.com/Articles/SAUNAS-NEAR%20VS.%20FAR%20I.htm

Craniosacral Therapy, 1983, John E Upledger, D.O., F.A.A.O. and Jon D. Vredevoogd, M.F.A

PEMF The 5th Element of Health, Bryant A. Meyers

Pulse Centers

Healing is Voltage, The Handbook, Jerry Tennant, MD, MD(H), PSc.,D

Chapter 8
Dr Angie Chaudoir-Ates ND, CNHP, CNC, MH Speaker at the DesBio 2016 Symposium, September 16th, 2016

http://www.naturalnews.com/045739_food_additives_FDA_toxic_chemicals.html

www.nongmoproject.org/gmo-facts/

http://restore4life.com/small-intestine/

http://articles.mercola.com/sites/articles/archive/2011/10/06/dangerous-toxins-from-gmo-foods.aspx

http://www.dailymail.co.uk/health/article-1388888/GM-food-toxins-blood-93-unborn-babies.html

http://articles.mercola.com/sites/articles/archive/2011/10/06/dangerous-toxins-from-gmo-foods.aspx

Digestive Wellness 4th Edition, Elizabeth Lipski, Ph.D., CCN, CHN

Dr. Donese Worden, NMD Speaker at DesBio 2016 Symposium, September 17th, 2017

Murakami K, Yoshino M, Aluminum decreases the glutathione regeneration by the inhibition of NADP-isocitrate dehydrogenase in mitochondria. Journal of Cellular Biochemistry. 2004 Dec 15; 93(6):1267-71

http://www.betterhealthguy.com/images/stories/PDF/kpu_klinghardt_explore_18-6.pdf

www.growyouthful.com/ailment/pyroluria.php

Chapter 9
Dr Lisa Holt, DAC, LAC, RN Speaker at DesBio 2016 Symposium, September 16th, 2016

The Beginner's Guide to Lyme Disease, Nicola McFadzean, N.D.

Healing Lyme Disease Coinfections, Stephen Harrod Buhner, 2013 pg

[10] Dr Myerowitz, D.C., Dilp. Ac. (NCCAOM), Lac., F.I.C.C., DABCA, BCIM speaker at the DesBio 2016 Symposium 9/17/2016

Chapter 10
Welcome to Morphogenic Field Technique Presented by Dr. Frank Springob, DC.

https://www.askdrmaxwell.com/2014/08/foods-that-make-you-hungry/

49728904R10067

Made in the USA
Columbia, SC
27 January 2019